MUSIC THERAPY

Learn How Music therapy Helps Depression, Stress and Mental Balance

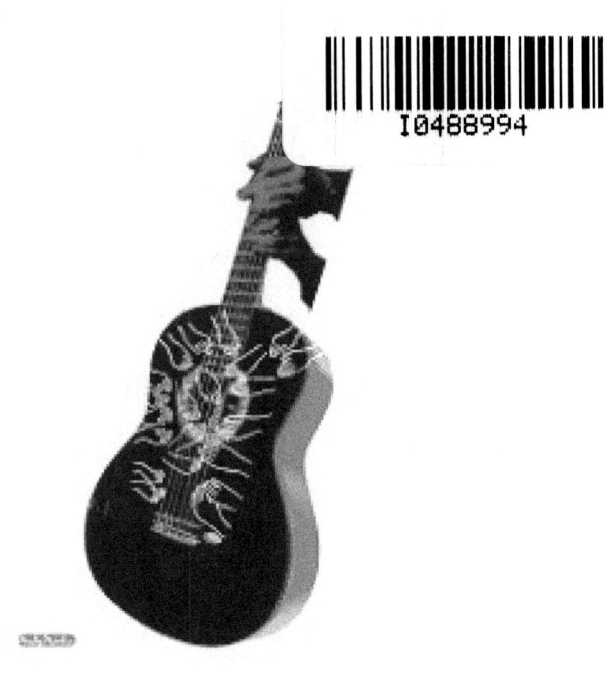

I0488994

By Patricia A Carlisle

Introduction

I want to thank you and congratulate you for choosing the book, *"MUSIC THERAPY: Learn How Music Therapy Helps Depression, Stress and Mental Balance"*.

Music is the food for the soul, for the earliest means of entertainment, worship and celebration music played a pivotal role in these areas still today, music continues to play a unique yet very important role in the entire universe. The sound of it dominates the earth and all human race bows to its rhythms. No one has been able to stop the diversification of music and music is so open ended that it continues to grow and bear different sounds which scientist have now notice that it could be explored for different purposes in all areas of life.

Hence, the subject matter, How Music Therapy Helps Depression, Stress and Mental Balance. Definitely, you will get to understand why the application of music therapy to a depressed and stressed mind can succeed in helping the individual maintain a psychological balance that will help the person raise a sigh of relief from his or her troubled mind. What then is music? How can it assist or work in the jurisdiction of a Therapist? Knowing that a therapist is from time to time visited with numerous health issues and only an expert can deliver a successful solution to issues concerning that kind or particular area that has to do with mental balance.

Thanks again for choosing this book, I hope you enjoy it!

ABOUT THE AUTHOR

Patricia A. Carlisle, MSW, CBT

Patricia Carlisle- a Master in Social Work and Cognitive Behavioral Therapist (CBT) gives out an expression of how important it is for an individual to take into consideration the concept of self-assessment to know what human, technical and conceptual skills they posses to perform or to achieve what they desire, or to deal with everyday life. However, every particular group of people has their own unique set of ideas, traditions and events including the frame of mind according to which people perform but there are many who faces problems and fail to maintain a healthy mind set affecting their behaviors and performance to those around them.

> People like Patricia Carlisle are among those who have felt this urge of serving people and helping them out of their mental crisis towards a healthy life. She has experienced some close encounters in her personal life regarding mental health issues in her family and friends that has encouraged her to pursue this as her career.

Currently Patricia Carlisle is serving as a Certified On-Line Cognitive Behavioral Therapist with an extensive 15years of experience using Cognitive-Behavior Therapy Techniques. She envisions a world where everyone gets mental health treatment with no mental health stigma and to make it real she has already set up her own Holistic Measure Online Comprehensive Behavioral Healthcare Company after retiring from The Nord Center in The Partial Hospitalization Program (PHP) Dept for 5 years and Murtis H. Taylor Mental Health Center as a mental health counselor, psychological support technician and case manager for 10 years to emulsify her skills more professionally.

Along with this, she has wrote down her passion as a clinician in 25 or more short books to help individuals and families get their life back, freeing them of the restraints of negative thinking, anxiety and depression by using different approaches. She is highly appreciated among her clients for her flexibility and professionalism of dealing with them graciously. To reach her, make use of her direct website address: http://therapist2013.wix.com/e-therapy . As she is ready to inspire hope and contribute to health and well-being by providing the best online health care through comprehensive practice, education and research.

TABLE OF CONTENT

Chapter 1

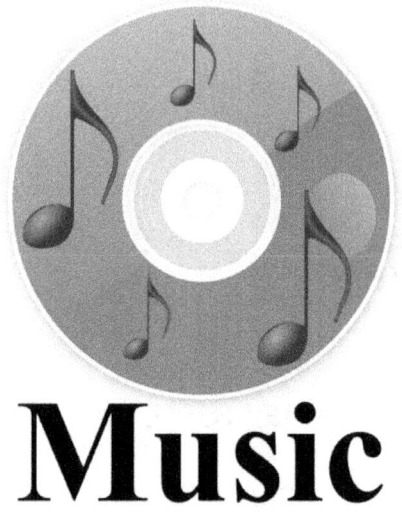

Music

MUSIC

Music is the science or art of ordering tones or sounds in succession, in combination and in temporal relationships to produce a composition having unity and continuity. A vocal, instrumental or mechanical sounds having rhythm, melody or harmony makes for the definition of music. There are also distinct types or categories of music.

The use of music in the earliest times was purely for entertainment and worship. That is why today we have so many worship songs that are used and administered in various religions of the world today; worship centers like; the churches, mosques, temple, etc. all make use of music in their order of procession and worship. Also worthy to note is the use of music by Christians, Muslims, Buddhist, cults, traditional religion and so many other groups who engage in the worship of a deity. It is a wide believe that we have a God or gods who we should worship as a supernatural being and who is in control of the universe, and the way and manner that form of worship will take place will include music most of the time.

USE OF MUSIC

Music used in Worship

Like we earlier said music is one of the earliest means of worshiping God through praises and hymns. The various religions around the world make use of music to worship God or gods in which they believe actually exist and who they feel is responsible for the control of the human race and the universe.

Music as a means of Entertainment

The world has seen a drastic divergence, sporadic, dynamic increase in technological and advanced development in the music sector both in the area of entertainment and industrially. Music in the entertainment sector has assumed a dimension that has catapulted the sector to a different level that was least expected to the extent that technology has really influenced music in a very big way. Highly advanced equipment has been produced, such that music can be and has been developed to one of the highest level of operation that continues to grow and develop in continuous advancement.

One of the areas that music has developed and its application has continued to generate a lot of interest is in the area of depression, stress and mental balance maintenance. Hence, the successful disposition of the human being in this area has seen how music has assisted in achieving a lot of success in its application to the lives of the troubled mind. When we talk about troubled mind, we are talking about those who are experiencing stress, depression and having an unbalanced mental status. In fact, the application of mental balance has a long way to go in most individual's life.

Without a balanced mental capability, there is no way an individual can function effectively both in the educational sector, work, employment or business sector. Therefore, much importance is placed on mental stability of an individual in the workplace or business organization. It will be a great disservice for any organization that has a workforce that comprises a huge risk for mental imbalance for their employees which should not be tolerated in any serious business organization.

Music in Sports Activities

The Olympics is one of the oldest sporting events where athletes comes from all corners of the world to compete for a Gold, Silver and bronze medal respectively. Music also forms part of the opening and closing ceremonies. Also in the events proper music are used as a means of entry, departure and special moments of victory. Not only in the Olympics other sporting activities like the FIFA World cup, European Champions Leagues and the Nations Cups are also events that are adorned with music.

Chapter 2

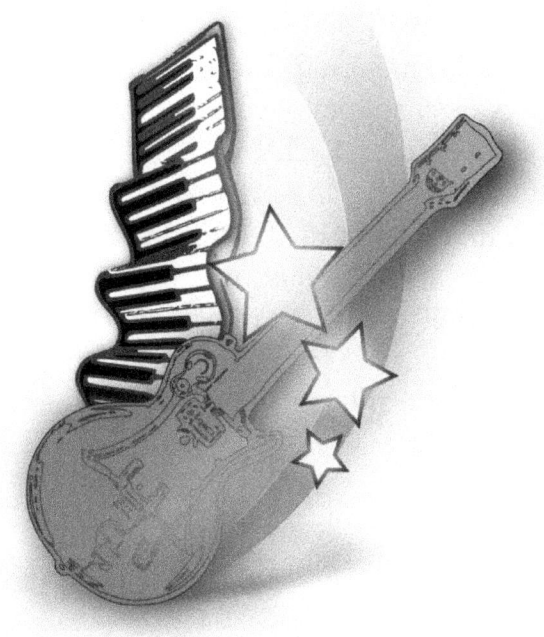

MUISC AS A THERAPY

If we are to look at the application of music as a mental health therapy, we look at how music relaxes our minds when the use of Music is administrated as a therapy. **So what then can be regarded as Music therapy?** Do you know that the use of music therapy is the administration of the use of music in interventions in order to accomplish a particular personal goal which exists in a therapeutic interconnection or relationship and it has to be done by a professional who has been successfully approved by or gone through a therapy programs.

Music therapist is a highly advanced health professional. In this regard the health professional who is involved in the administration of music which has to carry out the therapy in processes that is strictly approved and followed by a laid out procedure. It involves the use of therapy program which are physical, mental, emotional, social, spiritual and aesthetic to assist patients or clients to develop or improve their health in several platforms. Such as, cognitive therapists recommendation to clients to improve their health in diverse avenues, the functioning of their cognitive thinking capacity, motor skills, social skill, emotional growth advancement and generally the quality of life the individual is living or intends to live. Also, is responsible for further assistance in helping him or her to achieve the greatest benefit of the therapy the person is undergoing.

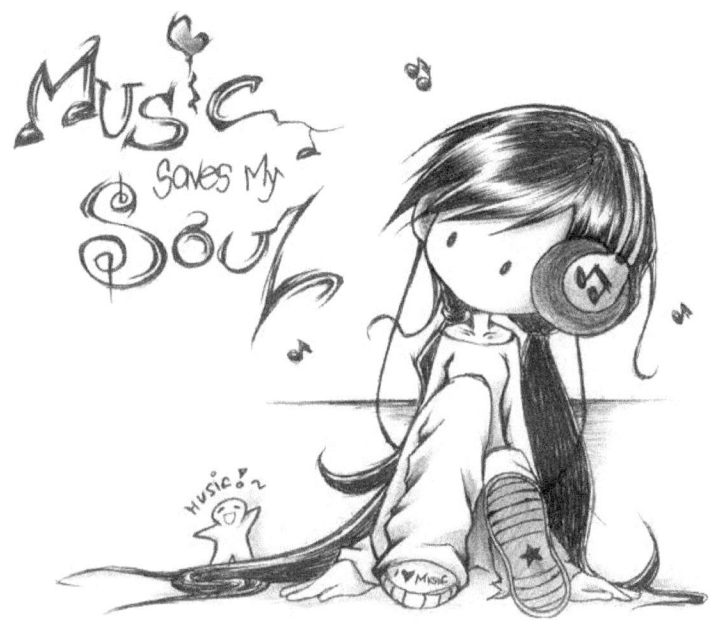

Chapter 3

ADMINISTRATION OF MUSIC THERAPY

The administration of music therapy such as singing, free improvisation, discussing, listening and moving to music to help reach treatment goals is very unique. It has a unique methodological approach which incorporates and makes use of clinical therapy, bi-musicology, music theory, musical acoustics, psychotherapy, psychoacoustics, aesthetic of music embodied music reasoning, comparative musicology and sensory integration; these methodologies are applied in every ramification to make sure that the individual suffering from mental depression or stress experiences that therapeutic nature that will enable him or her to get over what clouds their mind.

Depression or stress can cause a mental in-balance which leads to many adverse effects to an individual's perception, focus and concentration, and this can cause problems especially if they are a part of the workforce. Knowing that a large percentage of the working populations constitute the majority of active individuals in society which the government or private sector relies on to drive the economy or industries; the work force is responsible for the above undertakings and when they are hugely affected by circumstances that have to do with mental in-balance, there is a problem that needs to be addressed.

Both managers, directors of ministries and civil servants are not left out of the situation when faced with this kind of circumstances. Therefore referrals for music therapy services are suggested by other health care professionals such as psychologists, physicians, physical therapists and also the occupational therapists. Therefore, music therapists are available in almost every profession responsible for delivering healthcare services. It is only in some underdeveloped countries that have problems with availability of trained experts and personnel in that area who can deliver adequate solutions to the numerous problems that is associated with therapy in music. There is a huge gap in this area and which experts can take advantage by rendering skilled services in music therapy to online clients and customers who wish explore a career to learn music therapy so they can render the services locally.

Chapter 4

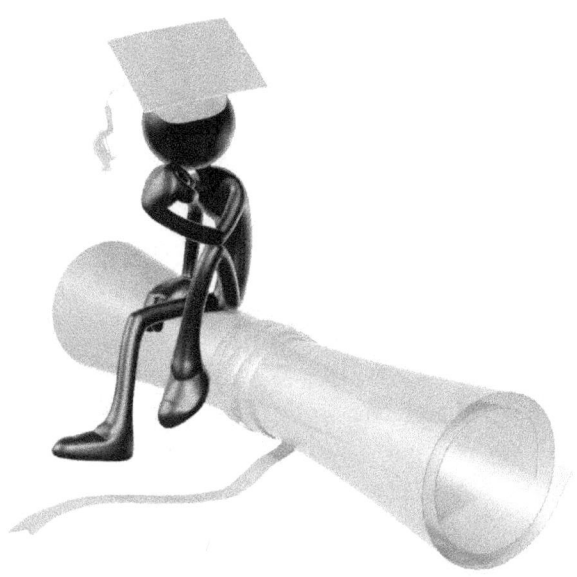

MUSIC THERAPIST COMMON PRACTICES

Music therapists assist other professionals in many ways, some common practices involves generating developmental work schedule which comprises of communication, motor skills for the persons with specific needs, also listening to reminiscence orientation music or song writing with an elderly mindset are also part of the process. This will also include rhythmic entertainment procedures to enhance rehabilitation of a sick or depressed person. The rhythmic entertainment for physical rehabilitation is applied for many depressed and problem ridden persons, for instance, persons who have had a stroke which is a medical condition that is linked to stress; music therapy can be administered in such situation. Some hospitals also use music therapy to administer at cancer centers as well.

FORMS MUSIC THERAPY

The use and Administration of Treatment using Music Therapy is divided into two different forms which are: **(a) active** and **(b) receptive** therapy methods respectively. When we make reference to the active music therapy we are talking about the situation where the therapist and the patient take active participation in creating music with the use of musical instruments, both parties, use their voice or other objects to carry out the therapy. This enables the patient to be creative and showcase or express his or herself through musical art.

While (b) receptive therapy is more of creating a relaxed setting where the therapist can play or make the music for the patient who is at liberty to listen, draw or meditate on the rhythms. This method brings a lot of therapeutic benefit to the patient when the individual's mind is drawn to the sounds and scenario of the music being played. It is the practice of the therapist to determine the method suitable to apply and the genre of music which is always in accordance with set rules and acceptable practice except unless specifically requested by the patient who feels he or she can choose the genre more suitable for his or her condition.

Chapter 5

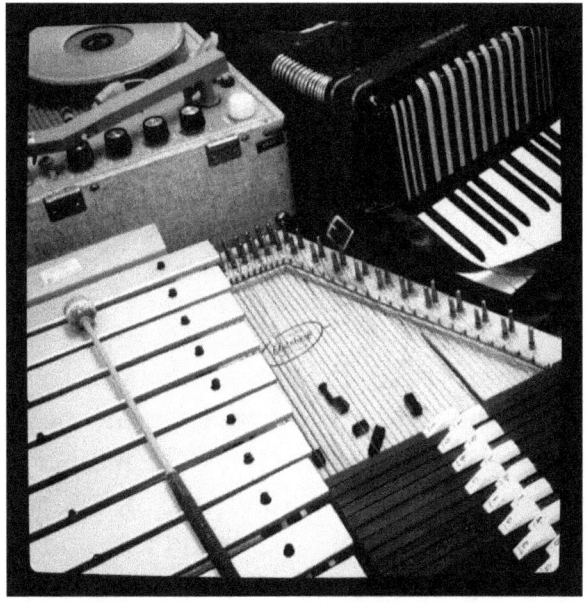

WHERE MUSIC THERAPY IS USED OR ADMINISTERED

Cancer Center

Music therapy is used in cancer centers during treatment of patients who are cancer ridden and suffering a great deal, music therapy helps them to get their mindset straight and helps them to stay positive to the true course of the treatment, if their mindset is hindered from the treatment, that could lead to further psychological problem that could disturb the treatment process all together.

Schools

Music therapy is administered in schools to assist the treatment and development of student with impairments and students who lack or have challenging problems which interferes with them studying effectively like the other students, such as, the physically challenge students. Also, students that appear to have no challenges with their mind are not left out of music therapy treatment, the therapy is also used in assisting them in the means of learning and maintaining a mental balance that helps them in focusing on their studies.

Baby Sitting

Music therapy is also used in helping a baby or a child sleep especially when the child is crying and irritated, or if the child is unable to sleep at night. Sometimes the mother engage the child in listening to music that will make the child feel sleepy thereby causing them to feel relaxed and the mother feel relief from the disturbances that the child is going through, when the relief is felt, the child finally goes back to sleep. You also have some mothers who sing love songs to their children to help them to fall asleep.

Conclusion

Thank you again for choosing this book!

I hope this book was able to help you to understand the benefits of music therapy.

Today music therapy is a continuous work in progress, there are various issues concerning music therapy which is yet to be exhausted, but we have taken time to do extensive research on some of the ordinary issues relating to it.

Psychological problems, neural-oriented problems and traumas can be taken care of to a large extent with the administration of music therapy which will always help and assist in the reduction of stress, depression and providing an acceptable mental balance needed for adequate development.

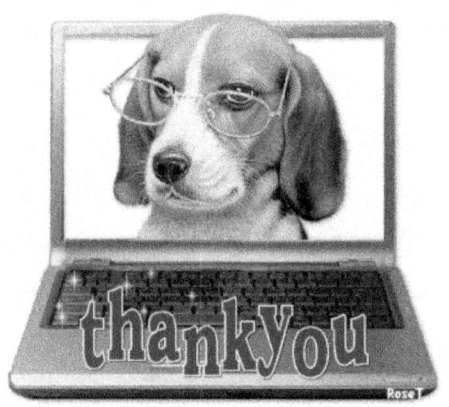

Finally, if you enjoyed this book, would you be kind enough to leave a review for this book on Amazon? It'd be greatly appreciated!

Thank you and good luck!

Preview Of 'PET THERAPY: Learn How To Use Pet Therapy To Control Your Mental Illness'

Chapter 1

PET THERAPY

Research shows that visiting with a pet can reduce stress symptoms, lower blood pressure temporarily, increase sensory stimulation, and even lengthen a person's life expectancy. Pet therapy is a general term that encompasses many therapeutic activities involving animals as companions or occasional visitors to the sick, elderly, or mentally ill. Because animals provide unconditional acceptance, pet therapy can be comforting and can also distract the sick or the aged from their illnesses or problems.

In areas that are often sterile and lonely, such as hospital or nursing homes, a pet therapy program can bring screened animals and human volunteers to make visits. These visits can be soothing the patients or residents, because people tend to be nurturing around animals. When participating in pet therapy, some patients recall fond memories about their own pets. These types of visits are shown to positively affect disposition and increase social interaction among patients and residents.

Other research has shown that heart patients who either own a pet or are paired with a pet following discharge from the hospital tend to heal faster and survive longer. Most likely this is due to the combination of a sense of purpose and the fact that having a pet can lower stress. The pet does not have to be a dog or cat; it can be a rabbit, fish, parakeet, or other animal.

Many pet therapy programs exist to train, coordinate, and place pets that have been behaviorally and medically screened in schools, medical centers, and homes for the elderly and troubled teenagers. Pet therapy can have a positive effect on a resident or patient's physical health, as well as on his or her emotional health by reducing loneliness and creating a sense of purpose.

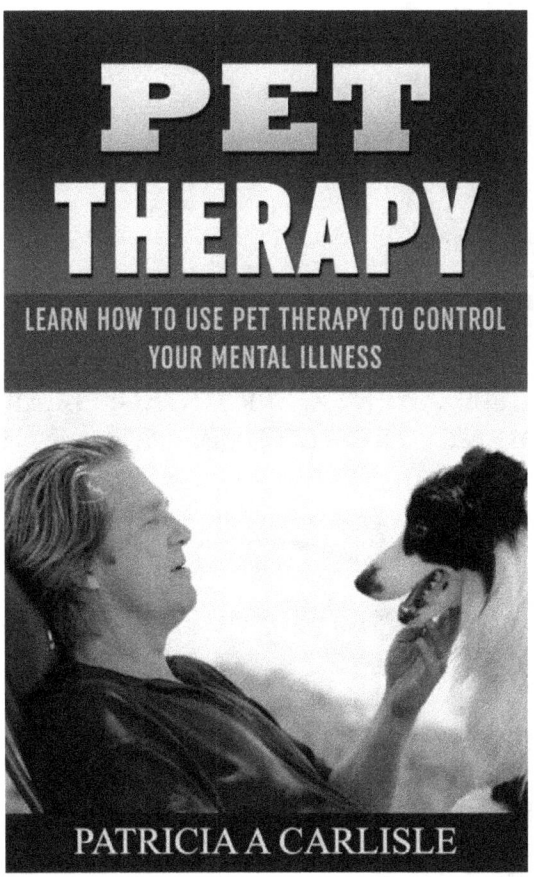

To check out the rest of (PET THERAPY: Learn How To Use Pet Therapy To control Your Mental Illness) go to Amazon.com.

Check Out My Other Books

Below you'll find some of my other popular books that are popular on Amazon and Kindle as well. Alternatively, you can visit my author page on Amazon to see other work done by me.

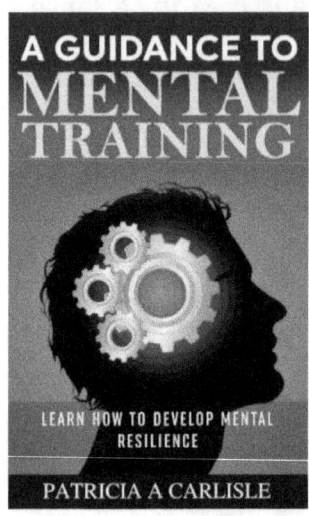

A GUIDANCE TO MENTAL TRAINING: LEARN HOW TO DEVELOP MENTAL RESILIENCE.

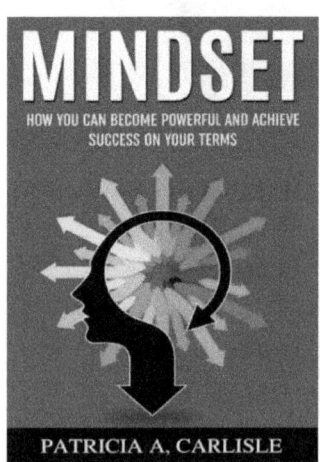

MINDSET: HOW YOU CAN BECOME POWERFUL AND ACHIEVE SUCCESS ON YOUR TERMS.

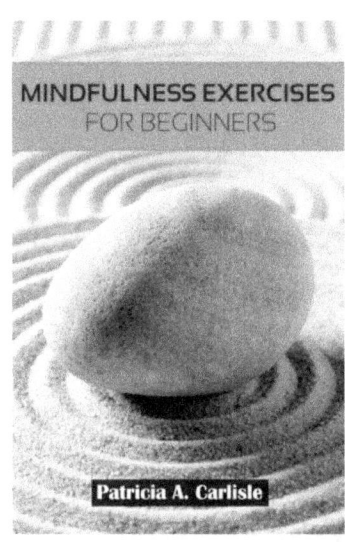

MINDFULNESS EXERCISES FOR BEGINNERS.

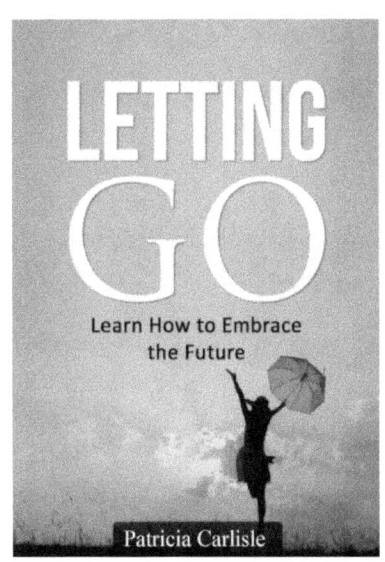

LETTING GO: LEARN HOW TO EMBRACE THE FUTURE.

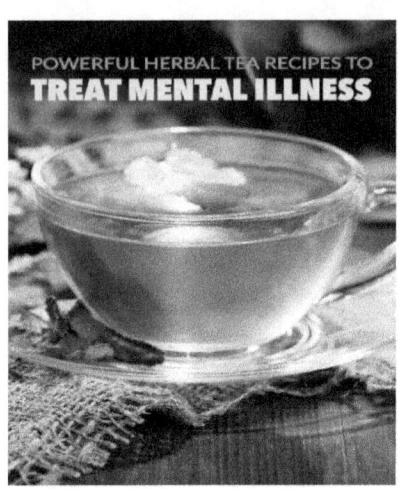

POWERFUL HERBAL TEA RECIPES TO TREAT MENTAL ILLNESS.

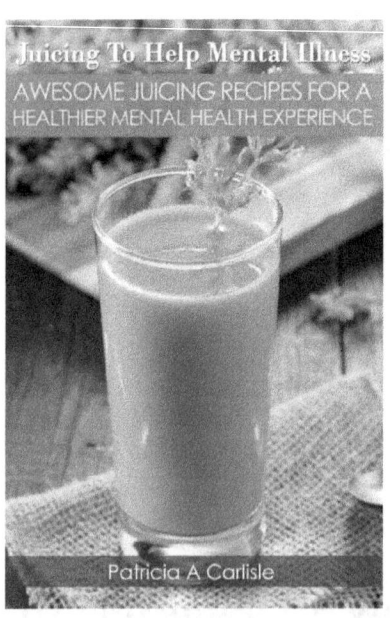

JUICING TO HELP MENTAL ILLNESS AWESOME JUICING RECIPES FOR A HEALTHER MENTAL HEATLH EXPERIENCE:

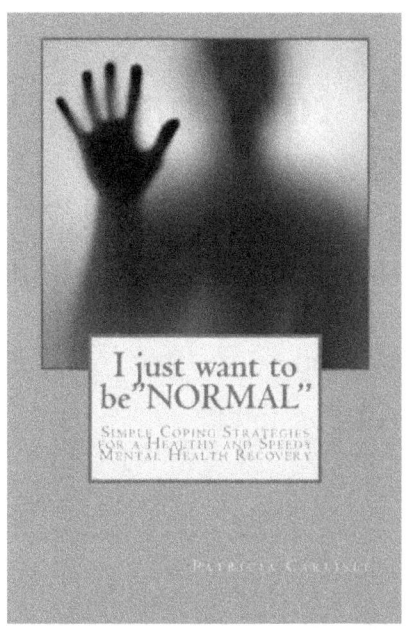

I Just want to be "NORMAL": Simple Coping Strategies for a Healthy and Speedy Mental Health Recovery.

You can simply search for these titles on the Amazon website to find them.

BONUS: SUBSCRIBE TO THE FREE BOOK

Beginners Guide to Yoga & Meditation

"Stressed out? Do You Feel Like The World Is Crashing Down Around You? Want To Take A Vacation That Will Relax Your Mind, Body And Spirit? Well this Easy To Read Step By Step

E-Book Makes It All Possible!"

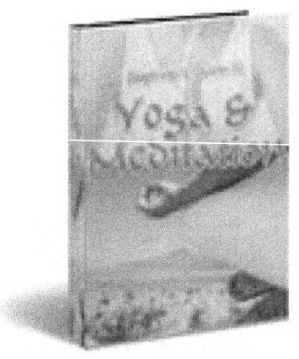

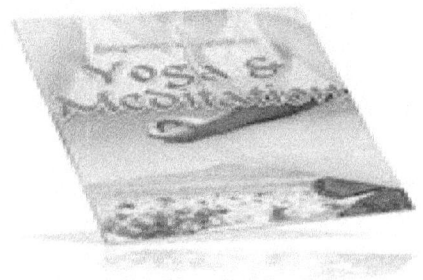

Instructions on how to join our mailing list, and receive a free copy of "Yoga and Meditation" can be found in any of my Kindle eBooks.

NOTES

NOTES

NOTES

NOTES

NOTES

NOTES

NOTES

NOTES

NOTES